Table of Contents

INTRODUCTION

An allergy is an immune system response to a foreign substance that's not typically harmful to your body. These foreign substances are called allergens. They can include certain foods, pollen, or pet dander. Your immune system's job is to keep you healthy by fighting harmful pathogens. It does this by attacking anything it thinks could put your body in danger. Depending on the allergen, this response may involve inflammation, sneezing, or a host of other symptoms. Your immune system normally adjusts to your environment. For example, when your body encounters something like pet dander, it should realize it's harmless. In people with dander allergies, the immune system perceives it as an outside invader threatening the body and attacks it. Allergies are common. Several treatments can help you avoid your symptoms.

Symptoms of allergies

The symptoms you experience because of allergies are the result of several factors. These include the type of allergy you have and how severe the allergy is. If you take any medication before an anticipated allergic response, you may still experience some of these symptoms, but they may be reduced.

For food allergies
Food allergies can trigger swelling, hives, nausea, fatigue, and more. It may take a while for a person to realize that they have a food allergy. If you have a serious reaction after a meal and you're not sure why, see a medical professional immediately. They can find the exact cause of your reaction or refer you to a specialist.

For seasonal allergies
Hay fever symptoms can mimic those of a cold. They include congestion, runny nose, and swollen eyes. Most of the time, you can manage these symptoms at home using over-the-counter

treatments. See your doctor if your symptoms become unmanageable.

For severe allergies
Severe allergies can cause anaphylaxis. This is a life-threatening emergency that can lead to breathing difficulties, lightheadedness, and loss of consciousness. If you're experiencing these symptoms after coming in contact with a possible allergen, seek medical help immediately. Everyone's signs and symptoms of an allergic reaction are different. Read more about allergy symptoms and what might cause them.

Allergies on skin

Skin allergies may be a sign or symptom of an allergy. They may also be the direct result of exposure to an allergen. For example, eating a food you're allergic to can cause several symptoms. You may experience tingling in your mouth and throat. You may also develop a rash. Contact dermatitis, however, is the result of your skin coming into direct contact with an allergen. This could happen if you touch something you're allergic to, such as a cleaning product or plant. Types of skin allergies include:

Rashes. Areas of skin are irritated, red, or swollen, and can be painful or itchy.

Eczema. Patches of skin become inflamed and can itch and bleed.

Contact dermatitis. Red, itchy patches of skin develop almost immediately after contact with an allergen.

Sore throat. Pharynx or throat is irritated or inflamed.

Hives. Red, itchy, and raised welts of various sizes and shapes develop on the surface of the skin.

Swollen eyes. Eyes may be watery or itchy and look "puffy."

Itching. There's irritation or inflammation in the skin.

Burning. Skin inflammation leads to discomfort and stinging sensations on the skin.

Rashes are one of the most common symptoms of a skin allergy. Find out how to identify rashes and how to treat them.

Causes of allergies

Researchers aren't exactly sure why the immune system causes an allergic reaction when a normally harmless foreign substance enters the body. Allergies have a genetic component. This means parents can pass them down to their children. However, only a general susceptibility to allergic reaction is genetic. Specific allergies aren't passed down. For instance, if your mother is allergic to shellfish, it doesn't necessarily mean that you'll be, too. Common types of allergens include:

Animal products. These include pet dander, dust mite waste, and cockroaches.

Drugs. Penicillin and sulfa drugs are common triggers.

Foods. Wheat, nuts, milk, shellfish, and egg allergies are common.

Insect stings. These include bees, wasps, and mosquitoes.

Mold. Airborne spores from mold can trigger a reaction.

Plants. Pollens from grass, weeds, and trees, as well as resin from plants such as poison ivy and poison oak, are very common plant allergens.

Other allergens. Latex, often found in latex gloves and condoms, and metals like nickel are also common allergens.

Seasonal allergies, also known as hay fever, are some of the most common allergies. These are caused by pollen released by plants. They cause:

itchy eyes

watery eyes

runny nose

coughing

Food allergies are becoming more common. Find out about the most common types of food allergies and the symptoms they cause.

Allergy treatments

The best way to avoid allergies is to stay away from whatever triggers the reaction. If that's not possible, there are treatment options available.

Medication

Allergy treatment often includes medications like antihistamines to control symptoms. The medication can be over the counter or prescription. What your doctor recommends depends on the severity of your allergies. Allergy medications include:

antihistamines like diphenhydramine (Benadryl)

corticosteroids

cetirizine (Zyrtec)

loratadine (Claritin)

cromolyn sodium (Gastrocrom)

decongestants (Afrin, Suphedrine PE, Sudafed)

leukotriene modifiers (Singulair, Zyflo)

Singulair should only be prescribed if there are no other suitable treatment options. This is because it increases your riskTrusted Source of serious behavioral and mood changes, such as suicidal thoughts and actions.

Immunotherapy

Many people opt for immunotherapy. This involves several injections over the course of a few years to help the body get used to your allergy. Successful immunotherapy can prevent allergy symptoms from returning.

Emergency epinephrine

If you have a severe, life-threatening allergy, carry an emergency epinephrine shot. The shot counters allergic reactions until medical help arrives. Common brands of this treatment include EpiPen and Twinject. Some allergic responses are a medical emergency. Prepare for these emergency situations by knowing allergic reaction first aid.

Natural remedies for allergies

Many natural remedies and supplements are marketed as a treatment and even a way to prevent allergies. Discuss these with your doctor before trying them. Some natural treatments may actually contain other allergens and make your symptoms worse. For example, some dried teas use flowers and plants that are closely related to plants that might be causing you serious sneezing. The same is true for essential oils. Some people use these oils to relieve common symptoms of allergies, but essential oils still contain ingredients that can cause allergies. The Each type of allergy has a host of natural remedies that may help speed up recovery. There are also natural options for children's allergies, too.

How allergies are diagnosed
Your doctor can diagnose allergies in several ways. First, your doctor will ask about your symptoms and perform a physical exam. They'll ask about anything unusual you may have eaten recently and any substances you may have come in contact with. For example, if you have a rash on your hands, your doctor may ask if you put on latex gloves recently. Lastly, a blood test and

skin test can confirm or diagnose allergens your doctor suspects you have.

Allergy blood test

Your doctor may order a blood test. Your blood will be tested for the presence of allergy-causing antibodies called immunoglobulin E (IgE). These are cells that react to allergens. Your doctor will use a blood test to confirm a diagnosis if they're worried about the potential for a severe allergic reaction.

Skin test

Your doctor may also refer you to an allergist for testing and treatment. A skin test is a common type of allergy test carried out by an allergist. During this test, your skin is pricked or scratched with small needles containing potential allergens. Your skin's reaction is documented. If you're allergic to a particular substance, your skin will become red and inflamed. Different tests may be needed to diagnose all your potential allergies. Start here to get a better understanding of how allergy testing works.

Preventing symptoms

There's no way to prevent allergies. But there are ways to prevent the symptoms from occurring. The best way to prevent allergy symptoms is to avoid the allergens that trigger them. The Avoidance is the most effective way to prevent food allergy symptoms. An elimination diet can help you determine the cause of your allergies so you know how to avoid them. To help you avoid food allergens, thoroughly read food labels and ask questions while dining out.

Preventing seasonal, contact, and other allergies comes down to knowing where the allergens are located and how to avoid them. If you're allergic to dust, for example, you can help reduce symptoms by installing proper air filters in your home, getting your air ducts professionally cleaned, and dusting your home regularly. Proper allergy testing can help you pinpoint your exact triggers, which makes them easier to avoid. These other tips can also help you avoid dangerous allergic reactions.

Complications of allergies

While you may think of allergies as those pesky sniffles and sneezes that come around every new season, some of these allergic reactions can actually be life-threatening. Anaphylaxis, for example, is a serious reaction to the exposure of allergens. Most people associate anaphylaxis with food, but any allergen can cause the telltale signs:

suddenly narrowed airways

increased heart rate

possible swelling of the tongue and mouth

Allergy symptoms can create many complications. Your doctor can help determine the cause of your symptoms as well as the difference between a sensitivity and a full-blown allergy. Your doctor can also teach you how to manage your allergy symptoms so that you can avoid the worst complications.

ASTHMA AND ALLERGIES

Asthma is a common respiratory condition. It makes breathing more difficult and can narrow the air passageways in your lungs. Asthma is closely related to allergies. Indeed, allergies can make existing asthma worse. It can also trigger asthma in a person who's never had the condition.

When these conditions occur together, it's a condition called allergy-induced asthma, or allergic asthma. Allergic asthma affects about 60 percent of people who have asthma in the United States, estimates the Allergy and Asthma Foundation of America. Many people with allergies may develop asthma. Here's how to recognize if it happens to you.

Allergies vs. cold

Runny nose, sneezing, and coughing are common symptoms of allergies. They also happen to be common symptoms of a cold and a sinus infection. Indeed, deciphering between the sometimes-generic symptoms can be difficult. However, additional signs and symptoms of the conditions may help you distinguish between the three. For example, allergies can cause rashes on your skin and itchy eyes. The common cold can lead to body aches, even fever. A sinus infection typically produces thick, yellow discharge from your nose. Allergies can impact your immune system for prolonged periods of time. When the immune system is compromised, it makes you more likely to pick up viruses you come into contact with. This includes the virus that causes the common cold. In turn, having allergies actually increases your risk for having more colds. Identify the differences between the two common conditions with this helpful chart.

Allergy cough

Hay fever can produce symptoms that include sneezing, coughing, and a persistent, stubborn cough. It's the result of your body's overreaction to allergens. It isn't contagious, but it can be miserable. Unlike a chronic cough, a cough caused by allergies and hay fever is temporary. You may only experience the symptoms of this seasonal allergy during specific times of the year, when plants are first blooming. Additionally, seasonal allergies can trigger asthma, and asthma can cause coughing. When a person with common seasonal allergies is exposed to an allergen, tightening airways can lead to a cough. Shortness of breath and chest tightening may also occur. Find out why hay fever coughs are typically worse at night and what you can do to ease them.

Allergies and bronchitis

Viruses or bacteria can cause bronchitis, or it can be the result of allergies. The first type, acute bronchitis, typically ends after several days or weeks. Chronic bronchitis, however, can linger for months, possibly longer. It may also return frequently. Exposure to common allergens is the most common cause of chronic bronchitis. These allergens include:

cigarette smoke

air pollution

dust

pollen

chemical fumes

Unlike seasonal allergies, many of these allergens linger in environments like houses or offices. That can make chronic bronchitis more persistent and more likely to return. A cough is the only common symptom between chronic and acute bronchitis. Learn the other symptoms of bronchitis so you can understand more clearly what you may have.

Allergies and babies

Skin allergies are more common in younger children today than they were just a few decades ago. However, skin allergies decrease as children grow older. Respiratory and food allergies become more common as children get older. Common skin allergies on babies include:

Eczema. This is an inflammatory skin condition that causes red rashes that itch. These rashes may develop slowly but be persistent.

Allergic contact dermatitis. This type of skin allergy appears quickly, often immediately after your baby comes into contact with the irritant. More serious contact dermatitis can develop into painful blisters and cause skin cracking.

Hives. Hives are red bumps or raised areas of skin that develop after exposure to an allergen. They don't become scaly and crack, but itching the hives may make the skin bleed.

Unusual rashes or hives on your baby's body may alarm you. Understanding the difference in the type of skin allergies babies commonly experience can help you find a better treatment.

Living with allergies

Allergies are common and don't have life-threatening consequences for most people. People who are at risk of anaphylaxis can learn how to manage their allergies and what to do in an emergency situation. Most allergies are manageable with avoidance, medications, and lifestyle changes. Working with your doctor or allergist can help reduce any major complications and make life more enjoyable.

SULFA ALLERGIES VS. SULFITE ALLERGIES

Despite having similar names and symptoms, sulfa and sulfite allergies are different. Sulfa refers to sulfonamides, known as sulfa drugs, while sulfite is commonly found in wine, processed food, and condiments. Sulfites and sulfa medications are chemically unrelated, but because their names are similar, people often confuse one with the other. Sulfa drugs were the first successful treatment against bacterial infections in the 1930s. They're still used today in antibiotics and other medications, like diuretics and anticonvulsants. People with HIV are at particular risk for sulfa sensitivity. Sulfites occur naturally in most wines. They're also used as a preservative in other foods.

Sulfa allergy

Symptoms of an allergic reaction to sulfa include:

hives

swelling of the face, mouth, tongue, and throat

drop in blood pressure

anaphylaxis (a severe, life threatening reaction that requires immediate medical attention)

Rarely, cases of serum sickness-like reactions can occur around 10 days after a sulfa drug treatment begins. Symptoms include:

fever

skin eruptions

hives

drug-induced arthritis

swollen lymph nodes

You should contact a doctor immediately if you have these symptoms.

Medications to avoid

Avoid the following medications if you're allergic or have a sensitivity to sulfa:

antibiotic combination drugs such as trimethoprim-sulfamethoxazole (Septra, Bactrim) and erythromycin-sulfisoxazole (Eryzole, Pediazole)

sulfasalazine (Azulfidine), which is used for Crohn's disease, ulcerative colitis, and rheumatoid arthritis

dapsone (Aczone), which is used to treat Hansen's disease (leprosy), dermatitis, and certain types of pneumonia

Safe medications for people with sulfa allergies

Not all drugs that contain sulfonamides cause reactions in all people. Many people with sulfa allergies and sensitivities may be able to safely take the following medications but should do so with caution:

some diabetes medications, including glyburide (Glynase, Diabeta) and glimepiride (Amaryl)

migraine medication sumatriptan (Imitrex, Sumavel, and Dosepro)

some diuretics, including hydrochlorothiazide (Microzide) and furosemide (Lasix)

The ability to take these medications can vary from person to person. If you have a sulfa allergy and are unsure if you should take any of these medications, talk with your doctor.

Sulfite allergy

Symptoms of an allergic reaction to sulfites include:

headache

rash

hives

swelling of the mouth and lips

wheezing or trouble breathing

asthma attack (in people with asthma)

anaphylaxis

If you experience more serious symptoms of a sulfite allergy, contact your doctor. Anaphylaxis requires emergency medical attention. According to the Cleveland Clinic, people with asthma have between a 1 in 20 and 1 in 100 chance of having a reaction to sulfites.

Sulfites are common in processed foods, condiments, and alcoholic beverages, such as red and white wine. Sulfites occur naturally in wine during fermentation, and many winemakers add them to help the process along. For the past two decades, the Food and Drug Administration (FDA) has required winemakers to display the warning "contains sulfites" if levels exceed a certain threshold. Many companies voluntarily add the label to their products as well. If you have sensitivities, you should avoid food products with the following chemicals on the label:

sulfur dioxide

potassium bisulfate

potassium metabisulfite

sodium bisulfite

sodium metabisulfite

sodium sulfite

Work with your doctor

Work with your doctor to determine the best course of action if you suspect you have a sulfa or sulfite allergy. You may need to see a specialist or undergo further testing. Be sure to talk to your doctor about which medications and products to avoid, especially if you have asthma.

THE 8 MOST COMMON FOOD INTOLERANCES

Food intolerance may cause symptoms similar to a food allergy in some people. These include diarrhea, bloating, and rashes. If you suspect you have a food intolerance, it's important to speak with a doctor. Unlike some allergies, food intolerances aren't life-threatening. However, they can be very problematic for those affected. Food intolerances and sensitivities are extremely common and seem to be on the rise. I In fact, it's estimated that up to 20% of the world's population may have a food intolerance. The Food intolerances and sensitivities can be hard to diagnose due to their wide range of symptoms.

What Is a Food Intolerance?

The term "food hypersensitivity" refers to both food allergies and food intolerances (3). A food intolerance is not the same as a food allergy, although some of the symptoms may be similar. In fact, it can be difficult to tell food allergies and food intolerances apart, making it important to speak with your doctor if you suspect you might have an intolerance. When you have a food intolerance, symptoms usually begin within a few hours of eating the food that you are intolerant to. Yet, symptoms can be delayed by up to 48 hours and last for hours or even days, making the offending food especially difficult to pinpoint. I What's more, if you frequently consume foods that you are intolerant to, it may be difficult to correlate symptoms to a specific food. While symptoms of food intolerances vary, they most often involve the digestive system, skin and respiratory system.Common symptoms include

Diarrhea

Bloating

Rashes

Headaches

Nausea

Fatigue

Abdominal

pain

Runny nose

Reflux

Flushing of the skin

Food intolerances are commonly diagnosed by elimination diets specifically designed to narrow down offending foods or through other testing methods. Elimination diets remove foods most commonly associated with intolerances for a period of time until symptoms subside. Foods are then reintroduced one at a time while monitoring for symptoms. The This type of diet helps people identify which food or foods are causing symptoms.

Here are 8 of the most common food intolerances.

1. Dairy

Lactose is a sugar found in milk and dairy products. It is broken down in the body by an enzyme called lactase, which is necessary in order for lactose to be properly digested and absorbed. Lactose intolerance is caused by a shortage of lactase enzymes, which causes an inability to digest lactose and results in digestive symptoms. Symptoms of lactose intolerance include:

Abdominal

pain

Bloating

Diarrhea

Gas

Nausea

Lactose intolerance is extremely common.

In fact, it is estimated that 65% of the world's population has trouble digesting lactose (8). Intolerance can be diagnosed several ways, including a lactose-tolerance test, lactose breath test or stool PH test. If you think you may have an intolerance to lactose, avoid dairy products that contain lactose, such as milk and ice cream.

Aged cheeses and fermented products like kefir may be easier for those with lactose intolerance to tolerate, as they contain less lactose than other dairy products and

Lactose intolerance is common and involves digestive symptoms including diarrhea, bloating and gas. People with lactose intolerance should avoid dairy products like milk and ice cream.

2. Gluten

Gluten is the general name given to proteins found in wheat, barley, rye and triticale.Several conditions relate to gluten, including celiac disease, non-celiac gluten sensitivity and wheat allergy. Celiac disease involves an immune response, which is why it is classified as an autoimmune disease. The When people with celiac disease are exposed to gluten, the immune system attacks the small intestine and can cause serious harm to the digestive system. Wheat allergies are often confused with celiac disease due to their similar symptoms.

They differ in that wheat allergies generate an allergy-producing antibody to proteins in wheat, while celiac disease is caused by an abnormal immune reaction to gluten in particular. The However, many people experience unpleasant symptoms even when they test negative for celiac disease or a wheat allergy. This is known as non-celiac gluten sensitivity, a milder form of gluten intolerance that has been estimated to impact anywhere from 0.5 to 13% of the population. Symptoms of non-celiac gluten sensitivity are similar to those of celiac disease and include:

Bloating

Abdominal

pain

Diarrhea

or constipation

Headaches

Fatigue

Joint pain

Skin rash

Depression

or anxiety

Anemia

Both celiac disease and non-celiac gluten sensitivity are managed with a gluten-free diet. It involves adhering to a diet free from foods and products that contain gluten, including:

Bread

Pasta

Cereals

Beer

Baked goods

Crackers

Sauces, dressing and gravies, especially soy sauce

Summary Gluten is a protein found in wheat,

barley, rye and triticale. People with an intolerance to gluten may experience

symptoms such as abdominal pain, bloating and headaches.

3. Caffeine

Caffeine is a bitter chemical that is found in a wide variety of beverages, including coffee, soda, tea and energy drinks. It's a stimulant, meaning it reduces fatigue and increases alertness when consumed. It does so by blocking receptors for adenosine, a neurotransmitter that regulates the sleep-wake cycle and causes drowsiness. The Most adults can safely consume up to 400 mg of caffeine a day without any side effects. This is the amount of caffeine in about four cups of coffee. The However, some people are more sensitive to caffeine and experience reactions even after consuming a small amount.

This hypersensitivity to caffeine has been linked to genetics, as well as a decreased ability to metabolize and excrete caffeine. The A caffeine sensitivity is different than a caffeine allergy, which involves the immune system. The People with a hypersensitivity to caffeine may experience the following symptoms after consuming even a small amount of caffeine:

Rapid

heartbeat

Anxiety

Jitters

Insomnia

Nervousness

Restlessness

People with a sensitivity to caffeine should minimize their intake by avoiding foods and beverages that contain caffeine, including coffee, soda, energy drinks, tea and chocolate.

Caffeine is a common stimulant to which some people are hypersensitive. Even a small amount can cause anxiety, rapid heartbeat and insomnia in some individuals.

4. Salicylates

Salicylates are natural chemicals that are produced by plants as a defense against environmental stressors like insects and disease Salicylates have anti-inflammatory properties. In fact, foods rich in these compounds have been shown to protect against certain diseases like colorectal cancer. The These natural chemicals are found in a wide range of foods, including fruits, vegetables, teas, coffee, spices, nuts and honey.Aside from being a natural component of many foods, salicylates are often used as a food preservative and may be found in medications. While excessive amounts of salicylates can cause health problems, most people have no problem consuming normal amounts of salicylates found in foods.

However, some people are extremely sensitive to these compounds and develop adverse reactions when they consume even small amounts. Symptoms of salicylate intolerance include:

Stuffy

nose

Sinus

infections

Nasal and

sinus polyps

Asthma

Diarrhea

Gut

inflammation (colitis)

Hives

While completely removing salicylates from the diet is impossible, those with a salicylate intolerance should avoid foods high in salicylates like spices, coffee, raisins and oranges, as well as cosmetics and medications that contain salicylates (20Trusted Source).

Salicylates are chemicals found naturally in many foods and used as preservatives in foods and medications. People who are intolerant to salicylates can experience symptoms like hives,

stuffy nose and diarrhea when exposed.

5. Amines

Amines are produced by bacteria during food storage and fermentation and found in a wide variety of foods. Though there are many types of amines, histamine is most frequently associated with food-related intolerance. Histamine is a chemical in the body that plays a role in the immune, digestive and nervous systems. It helps protect the body from infection by creating an immediate inflammatory response to allergens. This triggers sneezing, itching and watery eyes in order to potentially excrete harmful invaders. The In people without an intolerance, histamine is easily metabolized and excreted.

However, some people are not able to break down histamine properly, causing it to build up in the body. The most common reason for histamine intolerance is impaired function of the enzymes responsible for breaking down histamine — diamine oxidase and N-methyltransferase. The Symptoms of histamine intolerance include:

Flushing

of the skin

Headaches

Hives

Itching

Anxiety

Stomach

cramps

Diarrhea

Low blood pressure

People with an intolerance to histamine should avoid foods high in this natural chemical, including:

Fermented

foods

Cured

meats

Dried

fruits

Citrus

fruits

Avocados

Aged

cheeses

Smoked

fish

Vinegar

Soured

foods like buttermilk

Fermented alcoholic beverages like beer and wine

Summary Histamine is a compound that can cause

symptoms like itching, hives and stomach cramps in people who are unable to

properly break down and excrete it from the body.

6. FODMAPs

FODMAPs is an abbreviation that stands for fermentable oligo-, di-, mono-saccharides and polyols. I They are a group of short-chain carbohydrates found naturally in many foods that can cause digestive distress.

FODMAPs are poorly absorbed in the small intestine and travel to the large intestine, where they are used as fuel for the gut bacteria there. The bacteria break down or "ferment" the FODMAPs, which produces gas and causes bloating and discomfort. These carbohydrates also have osmotic properties, meaning they draw water into the digestive system, causing diarrhea and discomfort to Symptoms of a FODMAP intolerance include:

Bloating

Diarrhea

Gas

Abdominal

pain

Constipation

FODMAP intolerances are very common in people with irritable bowel syndrome, or IBS.In fact, up to 86% of people diagnosed with IBS experience a reduction in digestive symptoms when following a low-FODMAP diet. The There are many foods high in FODMAPs, including:

Apples

Soft

cheeses

Honey

Milk

Artichokes

Bread

Beans

Lentils

Beer

Summary FODMAPs are a group of short-chain

carbohydrates found in a wide array foods. They can cause digestive distress in

many people, especially those with IBS.

7. Sulfites

Sulfites are chemicals that are primarily used as preservatives in foods, drinks and some medications. They can also be found naturally in some foods like grapes and aged cheeses. Sulfites are added to foods like dried fruit to delay browning and wine to prevent spoilage caused by bacteria. The Most people can tolerate the sulfites found in foods and beverages, but some people are sensitive to these chemicals.Sulfite sensitivity is most common in people with asthma, though people without asthma can be intolerant to sulfites as well.Common symptoms of sulfite sensitivity include:

Hives

Swelling of the skin

Stuffy nose

Hypotension

Flushing

Diarrhea

Wheezing

Coughing

Sulfites can even cause airway constriction in asthmatic patients with sulfite sensitivity, and, in severe cases, it can lead to life-threatening reactions. The Food and Drug Administration (FDA) mandates that the use of sulfites must be declared on the label of any food that contains sulfites or where sulfites were used during the processing of food. The Examples of foods that may contain sulfites include:

Dried

fruit

Wine

Apple

cider

Canned

vegetables

Pickled

foods

Condiments

Potato

chips

Beer

Tea

Baked goods

Summary Sulfites are commonly used as

preservatives and can be found naturally in certain foods. People who are

hypersensitive to sulfites can experience symptoms like stuffy nose, wheezing

and low blood pressure.

8. Fructose

Fructose, which is a type of FODMAP, is a simple sugar found in fruits and vegetables, as well as sweeteners like honey, agave and high-fructose corn syrup. The consumption of fructose, especially from sugar-sweetened beverages, has risen dramatically in the past forty years and been linked to an increase in obesity, liver disease and heart disease. The Aside from a rise in fructose-related diseases, there has also been a surge in fructose malabsorption and intolerance. In people with fructose intolerance, fructose isn't efficiently absorbed into the blood. The Instead, the malabsorbed fructose travels to the large intestine, where it is fermented by gut bacteria, causing digestive distress and Symptoms of fructose malabsorption include:

Reflux

Gas

Diarrhea

Nausea

Abdominal

pain

Vomiting

Bloating

People with an intolerance to fructose are often also sensitive to other FODMAPs and can benefit from following a low-FODMAP diet.In order to manage symptoms related to fructose malabsorption, the following high-fructose foods should be avoided:

Soda

Honey

Apples,

apple juice and apple cider

Agave

nectar

Foods

containing high-fructose corn syrup

Certain

fruits like watermelon, cherries and pears

Certain vegetables like sugar snap peas

Summary Fructose is a simple sugar that is

malabsorbed by many people. It can cause symptoms such as bloating, gas and

diarrhea in those who can't properly absorb it.

Other Common Food Intolerances
The food intolerances listed above are among the most common types. However, there are many other foods and ingredients to which people may be intolerant, including:

Aspartame: Aspartame is an artificial sweetener that is commonly used as a sugar substitute. Although research is conflicting, some studies have reported

side effects like depression and irritability in people with a sensitivity

(37Trusted Source).

Eggs: Some people have difficulty

digesting egg whites but are not allergic to eggs. Egg intolerance is associated with

symptoms like diarrhea and abdominal pain (38Trusted Source).

MSG: Monosodium glutamate, or MSG, is used as a flavor-enhancing additive in foods. More research is needed, but some studies have shown that large

amounts can cause headache, hives and chest pain (39Trusted Source, 40Trusted Source).

Food colorings: Food colorings like Red 40 and Yellow 5 have been shown to

cause hypersensitivity reactions in some people. Symptoms include hives,

skin swelling and stuffy nose (41).

Yeast: People with a yeast intolerance generally experience less severe symptoms than those with a yeast allergy.

Symptoms are typically limited to the digestive system.

Sugar alcohols: Sugar alcohols are often used as zero calorie alternatives

to sugar. They can cause major digestive issues in some people, including;

bloating and diarrhea

Summary There are many foods and food additives

to which people are intolerant. Food colorings, MSG, eggs, aspartame and sugar

alcohols have all been shown to cause symptoms in certain people.

Food intolerances differ from allergies. Most do not trigger the immune system, and their symptoms are usually less severe. However, they can negatively impact your health and should be taken seriously. Many people are intolerant or hypersensitive to foods and additives like dairy products, caffeine and gluten. If you suspect that you may be intolerant to a certain food or food additive, speak to your doctor or dietitian about testing and treatment options.

Although food intolerances are usually less serious than food allergies, they can negatively affect your quality of life. This is why it's important to take steps to identify food intolerances in order to prevent unwanted symptoms and health issues.

Everything You Should Know If You're Considering Allergy Shots

Allergen immunotherapy consists of a series of treatments aimed at providing long-term relief from severe allergies. It's also known as:

allergy immunotherapy

subcutaneous immunotherapy

allergy shots

You might consider allergy shots if you have severe allergy symptoms that interfere with your daily life, even after you've made changes to your immediate environment. These shots may be used to treat allergies caused by:

dust mites

feathers

mold spores

pet dander, such as the kind from a cat or dog

pollen

stinging insects

When taken in the recommended sequence, allergy shots can provide significant symptom relief. At the same time, this treatment option requires a long-term commitment to work effectively.

Who's a good candidate for allergy shots?

This treatment method requires frequent injections at the doctor's office. You need to be able to commit time to it. Allergy shots may be used by people who have:

allergic asthma

allergic rhinitis

eye allergies, or allergic conjunctivitis

allergies to insects, particularly bees and other stinging insects

Allergy shots tend to work best for people who are sensitive to insect venoms and inhaled allergens. They are You may also be a good candidate if you experience severe allergy symptoms year-round and you don't want to take medications over a long period of time.

Who shouldn't take allergy shots?
Allergy shots are only used in people who are at least 5 years old. That's because children younger than 5 years old may not be able to fully communicate about potential side effects and

discomfort that would warrant stopping treatment. Allergy shots also aren't recommended if you:

are pregnant

have heart disease

have severe asthma

How do allergy shots work?

Allergy shots work by decreasing symptoms from particular allergens. Each injection contains small amounts of the allergen so that your body builds up immunity to it over time. The process works much like taking a vaccine, where your body creates new antibodies to combat the invasive substances.Allergy shots also improve the way other immune system cells and substances function in response to allergens. Eventually, successful immunotherapy helps the body fight off allergens and reduce adverse symptoms. Allergy shots aim to decrease overall allergy symptoms over time. If you have allergic asthma, reduced asthma symptoms are also possible.

How do you prepare for an allergy shot?

Before you start allergy shots, you'll need a full evaluation. The doctor needs to test your allergies to know exactly which substances to use in the shots. For example, if you have allergies during pollen season, they'll test for which types of pollen cause your symptoms. Ragweed, grasses, and various tree pollens are common culprits.

Allergy testing usually consists of skin pricking. During a skin prick test, your doctor will prick the skin on your back or forearm with several types of allergens to determine which ones cause reactions. A type of specialist known as an allergist or an immunologist will conduct all testing and treatment with allergy shots.

What's the procedure for an allergy shot?

Once your doctor has identified your allergens, you'll start receiving allergy shots. The process is broken down into two phases:

buildup

maintenance

Buildup

The buildup phase requires the largest time commitment. You receive injections up to twice per week to help your body get used to the allergens. You'll need to stay at your doctor's office for 30 minutes after each injection so they can monitor any side effects and reactions. The buildup phase typically lasts 3 to 6 months.

Maintenance

The maintenance phase consists of shots administered once or twice per month. You enter the maintenance phase once your doctor determines that your body has grown accustomed to the injections. They base this decision on your reaction to the shots. The maintenance phase typically lasts between 3 and 5 years. It's important that you don't skip any of your injections, if possible. Doing so can disrupt your treatment course. During this phase, you'll also need to stay at your doctor's office for 30 minutes post-injection so that they can monitor your reaction.

Are allergy shots effective?
Allergy shots can provide long-term relief well after the injections have stopped. The Some people who have received allergy shots may no longer need medication for their allergies.

However, it can take up to 1 year of maintenance shots before you see results. Some people may notice benefits early on in the maintenance phase, though. In some cases, allergy shots don't work. This may be due to a variety of reasons, including:

stopping treatment due to reactions

continued exposure to allergens at extremely high levels

not enough allergen in the actual shots

missed allergens during your initial evaluation

What are the side effects of allergy shots?

Common side effects include reactions that look like hives or mosquito bites at the site of the injection. The area can also swell to a larger bump and increase in redness. This type of reaction is normal. It can happen immediately or several hours after the injection.

It can last for several hours before going away without any treatment. You can help reduce swelling by applying ice to the injection site. Some people experience mild allergy symptoms — including nasal congestion, sneezing, and itchy skin — after their shots. This is a reaction to the allergens being injected. Taking an antihistamine can help ease these symptoms.

Rare side effects

In rare cases, allergy shots may cause a severe reaction, including:

hives

swelling

anaphylaxis

If you go into anaphylactic shock, you may experience dizziness and breathing difficulties. This reaction can develop within 30 minutes of receiving an allergy shot. This is why your doctor will likely ask you to stay at the office after the injection so that they can monitor you.

When you're feeling sick

If you're sick, let your doctor know. You may need to skip an injection until you've recovered. Taking an allergy shot while you have a respiratory illness, for example, could increase your risk for side effects.

How much do allergy shots cost?

Health insurance typically covers allergy shots. You may have to pay a copay for each visit. Copays are usually nominal fees. If you don't have health insurance, have a high deductible, or if allergy shots aren't covered under your plan, you may end up spending thousands of dollars a year. One large 2019 study looked at the costs of allergy shots for people with commercial insurance or Medicare Advantage with Part D. Researchers examined data gathered between 2013 and 2015.

The cost of allergy shots for 131,493 people totaled $253,301,575. This averages out to around $1,926 per person.

People with allergies covered about 19 percent of the total costs, while insurers covered about 81 percent.

On average, treatment lasted 463.1 days (or around 15 months).

Before beginning any treatment, talk with your doctor about payment options and costs.

Keep in mind that allergy shots are a long-term commitment. They require many injections, so you'll want to plan accordingly if you're paying out of pocket. Also consider that, over time, allergy shots could save you money on sick visits and over-the-counter (OTC) allergy medications.

EVERYTHING YOU NEED TO KNOW ABOUT RED MEAT ALLERGIES

Red meat isn't one of the top eight major food allergens, and an allergy to this food is a rather new discovery. But it's on the rise. In the United States, red meat allergies were first reported in 2009 with 24 cases. As of 2021, the number increased to 34,000 confirmed cases. Specifically, there was a 32% increase in cases of this allergy in the southeastern United States, where Lone Star ticks are common. These insects' bites may trigger red meat allergies. Currently, it's estimated that up to 3% of people in the United States are allergic to red meat.

What causes a red meat allergy?

Some evidenceTrusted Source suggests that red meat allergy in the United States may be triggered by tick bites, specifically from Lone Star ticks. Other tick species have been linked to this allergy in other countries. Although people of all ages can develop this allergy, most cases have been reported in adults who have been bitten by ticks. A tick bite may trigger an immune response to galactose-alpha-1,3-galactose (also known as alpha-gal), a sugar that's found in mammalian red meat, which humans tend to eat.

Alpha-gal reactions are recognized as a common cause of allergic reactions to red meat. It's also possible, though rare, to have a red meat allergy unrelated to alpha-gal syndrome. Not everyone who gets bitten by a Lone Star tick will develop an allergy. More research is needed to understand how ticks may trigger this reaction and what the risk factors are for its development. (In case you're wondering whether Lyme disease — another well-knownTrusted Source tick-borne disease — causes red meat allergies, no evidence suggests that the two conditions are related.)

Red meat allergy and COVID vaccines

You may be concerned about red meat allergies and the COVID-19 vaccine. The mRNA vaccines do not contain animal materials, which means their ingredients do not contain alpha-gal. The Centers for Disease Control and Prevention recommendsTrusted

Source that people who have had allergic reactions unrelated to the ingredients in the COVID-19 vaccine receive the vaccination. If you have concerns about your allergies and the COVID-19 vaccine, consult a healthcare professional.

What are the symptoms of a red meat allergy?
Symptoms of a red meat allergy can include:

hives or an itchy rash

digestive upset such as nausea, vomiting, heartburn, indigestion, diarrhea, and severe stomach pain

difficulty swallowing

swelling of lips, throat, tongue, or eyelids

dizziness or faintness

a drop in blood pressure

shortness of breath or difficulty breathing

Alpha-gal syndrome is unique in that symptoms do not begin until 3 to 6 hoursTrusted Source after eating red meat or dairy byproducts or after exposure to products that contain alpha-gal. Often, it can take longer. In contrast, symptoms of other food allergies, such as hives, vomiting, and difficulty breathing, typically start within 2 hours of eating the food. Symptoms and severity vary from person to person, and you may not have the same reaction with each exposure. If you experience difficulty breathing at any time, go to the nearest emergency room.

How is a red meat allergy diagnosed?

An allergist can diagnose red meat allergy through a detailed history consistent with alpha-gal type allergy. Healthcare professionals can confirm suspected alpha-gal syndrome with a blood test showing sensitization to alpha-gal. They may also use a blood test showing sensitization to mammalian meats. Additionally, an allergy skin test documenting reactions to red meat may be useful.

What treatment options are available for a red meat allergy?

If you have a red meat allergy, the only treatment is to limit or avoid red meat. If alpha-gal syndrome is the cause of your allergy, you may also need to limit or avoid foods that contain alpha-gal.

Alpha-gal can be foundTrusted Source in:

mammalian meats, including pork, beef, rabbit, lamb, and venison (organ meats have more alpha-gal than other cuts)

other products made from mammals, including gelatin, dairy, lard, tallow, suet, meat broth, bouillon, stock, and gravy

Rocky Mountain or prairie oysters (which are bull testicles, not real oysters)

Alpha-gal is notTrusted Source found in poultry — such as chicken, turkey, duck, and quail — or other birds. There is also no alpha-gal in eggs, fish and seafood, or reptiles. Keep in mind that red meat allergy differs for everyone. Some people may be able to eat small portions of foods containing allergens without experiencing symptoms, while others cannot. For example, most people with red meat allergies can tolerate cow's milk.

Remember to read the ingredient lists of products and medications. Ingredients that contain alpha-gal include gelatin, glycerin, magnesium stearate, and bovine extract. If you're limiting or avoiding red meat, be sure to replace it with poultry, eggs, seafood, or plant proteins to ensure that you're still following a balanced diet. Your diet can also include soy, pulses, nuts, seeds, and whole grains, none of which contain alpha-gal.

Is it possible to prevent a red meat allergy?
You can reduce your risk of developing red meat allergy caused by alpha-gal syndrome by preventing tick bites. Before you go outdoors, consider the following tips:

Know where to expect ticks. They usually reside in wooded, grassy, or brushy areas.

Treat clothing and gear with products containing 0.5% permethrin. You can also buy products that are pretreated.

Use Environmental Protection Agency-registered insect repellents.

You can minimize contact with ticks when you're outdoors by avoiding wooded and brushy areas and wearing long pants and closed-toed shoes with socks. Walk in the center of the trails, if possible. When you return from the outdoors:

Check your whole body for ticks. Pay special attention to your underarms, in and around your ears, inside your belly button, the backs of your knees, around your waist, your pubic area, and your hair. Here's how to remove a tick from your body if you find one.

Inspect your clothing. Remove any ticks you find on clothes, wash the clothes, and dry them on high heat for at least 10 minutes.

Examine your pets and gear for ticks.

Shower within 2 hours of coming indoors.

Other frequently asked questions

Does red meat allergy go away?

To date, there are no reports of a red meat allergy going away. However, there's emerging evidence that alpha-gal syndrome may subside over 1 to 5 yearsTrusted Source in most people.

How do you test for red meat intolerance?

Remember: An intolerance is different from an allergy. Allergies can affect your digestive system. However, an allergy is due to your immune system's hypersensitivity to an allergen. This reaction produces hives, vomiting, and other symptoms. Diarrhea and bloating are less common symptoms. Intolerance is not specifically due to your immune system, and digestive symptoms are its most common manifestations. An allergist will likely take a thorough medical history, perform a physical examination, and order a blood test to rule out an allergy. An allergy skin test may also be necessary. If you don't have an allergy, you may have an intolerance. There is no way to test for an intolerance besides monitoring your food intake and symptoms.

Red meat allergies are on the rise. Based on current evidence, alpha-gal syndrome, which is triggered by Lone Star tick bites in the United States, is a common cause. You can't treat or reverse a red meat allergy, but you can limit or stop red meat consumption to prevent symptoms. If you have alpha-gal syndrome, you may also need to avoid byproducts of red meat, although dairy is typically well tolerated. There's still a lot we don't know about the causes, treatment, and duration of red meat allergies. Consult a healthcare professional if you think you've been bitten by a Lone Star tick, especially if you develop any symptoms after a bite.

ALL ABOUT FOOD ALLERGY RASHES

More than 50 million Americans have an allergy of some kind. Food Allergy Research and Education (FARE) estimates up to 15 million people in the United States have a food allergy. A rash is one of several common symptoms that can occur if you have an allergic reaction to a food. Keep reading to learn more about what food rashes may look like and what you can do about them.

Signs of a food allergy rash

Food allergy reactions don't always include rashes. However, rashes associated with food allergies have symptoms such as:

hives

redness

itchiness

swelling

A rash tends to develop shortly after coming into contact with the food. With a food sensitivity it may appear around your mouth, neck, or face — basically anywhere food has come into contact with your skin. It's also possible to have a rash on other parts of your body. This is more common with a food allergy. Overall, the symptoms of a food allergy rash are the same among children and adults. You may be able to tell your rash is from a food allergy if you also have other symptoms of a food allergy, such as:

abdominal cramps

diarrhea

itchy or watery eyes

itchy, stuffy nose

sneezing

vomiting

Food allergy rash causes

Food allergy rashes are caused by ingesting foods you're allergic to. Your immune system treats the proteins in the food as harmful substances and tries to fight them. Even trace amounts can lead to an allergic reaction. According to the American Academy of Allergy, Asthma, and Immunology (AAAAI), the most common food allergens include:

cow's milk

eggs

fish

nuts

peanuts

shellfish

soy

wheat

While these are the most common, it's possible to be allergic to any food. In fact, FARE estimates that at least 170 foods can cause allergies. There's also the possibility of cross-reactivity. For example, if you're allergic to ragweed, you could also be allergic to foods in the same family, such as melons. A common cross-reactive allergy is latex and foods. People with latex allergies may also be allergic to fruits including bananas, kiwi, and avocado.

Food allergies are often detected during early childhood as a result of an adverse reaction to a particular food. Blood or skin tests can also help diagnose food allergies. Many children outgrow food allergies, but it's possible to have lifelong allergies. Adults can also develop new food allergies, though this is less common. The only way to avoid an allergic reaction is to avoid a food allergen entirely. While food labels are very important, it's also important for you to be prepared in case of a reaction.

Food allergy rash treatment

Food allergy rashes eventually subside once the underlying reaction stops. One of the best ways to help is to stop your exposure to the allergen.

Wash up

Wash your hands and face, if needed, as well as any surfaces that may have come in contact with the suspected food. This can help prevent more rashes. Some people rinse off with a quick shower.

Apply a soothing cream or gel

If the rash is bothersome, you can apply over-the-counter (OTC) creams, such as hydrocortisone.

Take an antihistamine

An oral antihistamine can also help. These will help alleviate the itchiness, inflammation, and overall discomfort. There are different OTC antihistamines, each with a different active ingredient. Some may work better than others for you and your symptoms. It takes time for the antihistamine to build up in your system. You shouldn't mix antihistamines. Take one type of antihistamine as directed while your rash is present.

Speak to a doctor

For your long-term health and comfort, it can be helpful to consult an allergist or even a nutritionist or dietitian. An allergist can help you to identify your allergens and determine what OTC antihistamine is appropriate for you. In addition, a nutritionist or dietitian can provide you with useful tips and suggestions for foods so you avoid your allergy trigger while still getting the right nutrition.

How long does a food allergy rash last?

A food allergy rash may not appear until your immune system reacts to the food. Depending on the food and the amount you ingest, this can take a few hours. Other cases can develop within minutes. Scratching at it can make it last longer. This can also increase your risk for skin infection.

Once your immune system calms down, your symptoms will subside. Antihistamines and topical creams can help alleviate minor symptoms. Overall, the rash should subside within a day or two. According to FARE, it's possible to have a second wave of food allergy symptoms, which may occur up to four hours after the initial reaction, though this is rare. Call your doctor if you think your initial food allergy rash has become infected. Signs may include inflammation, pain, and discharge. The size of the rash can also increase if it's infected.

Food allergy rash and anaphylaxis

The most severe type of allergic reaction is anaphylaxis, which is a life-threatening condition. This is not a complication of a food rash itself, but rather a complication of the overall allergic reaction. Hives and anaphylactic reactions often occur together, but you can have hives without having anaphylaxis. On top of the food allergy symptoms listed above, anaphylaxis may cause:

breathing difficulties

chest pain

dizziness

fainting

low blood pressure

severe swelling in the mouth, face, neck, and throat

tightness in the throat

tingling lips, hands, and feet

wheezing

If your doctor recommends epinephrine shots for severe food allergies, it's important to keep them on hand at all times. Even breathing in a food allergen can cause severe issues. Also, the severity of a reaction may vary — just because one reaction was mild, doesn't mean the next will also be mild.

Anaphylaxis is a medical emergency. Call 911 or your local emergency services and take your epinephrine shot as soon as you experience symptoms. Antihistamines can't treat anaphylaxis because the symptoms are too severe at this stage.

Food allergy rash vs. food intolerance

A food allergy occurs when your immune system adversely reacts to proteins in a certain food you're allergic to. This is not the same thing as a food intolerance. Food intolerance is primarily a digestive issue that can cause symptoms similar to food allergies, except that it's not life-threatening. Non-itchy rashes from a food intolerance can also develop over time, such as "chicken skin" on arms. This is unlike a food allergy rash, which tends to occur within minutes or hours of eating the suspected food. Food intolerance can also cause bloating, stomach pain, and mild digestive upset.

Another key difference is that you can sometimes have small amounts of a food without a problem if you have an intolerance. With an allergy, even a small amount of the food can cause issues.nAccording to the AAAAI, most suspected cases of food allergies are actually intolerances. However, you don't want to take a chance with self-diagnosis. An allergist can help you determine the difference.

CONCLUSION

If you suspect moderate to severe food allergies, make an appointment with an allergist. This type of specialist can accurately diagnose food allergies and rule out any possible food sensitivities. Since there's no cure for food allergies, the best way to prevent them — and subsequent symptoms like rashes — is to avoid the culprit completely.

9 7 9 8 8 7 2 3 6 9 2 1 9